# CAREER AS A
# CERTIFIED
# MEDICAL ASSISTANT

CHANCES ARE YOU ENCOUNTERED A medical assistant the last time you visited a physician. It could have been the person who scheduled your appointment, or whom you first met with in the exam room, asking routine questions while checking your vital signs. A medical assistant may have helped you with your bill or your prescription needs by calling or emailing the prescription into the pharmacist. Medical assistants are there to make sure you receive the best treatment possible.

There are many opportunities for employment in today's healthcare without undergoing the cost and training required to become a physician or nurse. A career as a certified medical assistant (CMA) stands out as an increasingly vital component in medical practice. Multi-skilled and versatile, medical assistants help care for people and improve productivity in a medical practice, while providing a human touch.

Along with the numerous scientific advances that have occurred in medical care over the past century, many changes have also taken place in the way medical care is provided. Long gone are the private practitioners, who until the 1970s often made house calls. These dedicated physicians provided individual care and typically were aided by only a single nurse and sometimes a secretary in the office (although the nurse often handled those duties).

With the introduction of managed care and other changes in the economics of healthcare, individual physician practices are disappearing. In their place are larger practices that typically include several doctors and a significant nursing and administrative staff. As a result, physician practices, from those focusing on general care, to specialists such as orthopedic surgeons and ophthalmologists, are turning to medical assistants in the interest of cost-effectiveness and efficiency. From assisting in running the office administratively to interacting with patients and helping with basic medical care, medical assistants with their wide range of skills are increasingly viewed as vital partners in caring for patients efficiently and effectively.

Because of the growing importance of medical assistants, more employers are requiring that their medical assistants be certified. Certification is acquired through the American Association of Medical Assistants, and reflects the field's growing professional status. The preparation for certification prepares a medical assistant for working in the real world.

It is important to point out that medical assistants are not the same as physician assistants (PAs). Although the scope of their work can vary according to state laws, PAs typically do not perform administrative functions but focus their efforts on therapeutic and preventive healthcare. They often work more independently than the medical assistant and, under the supervision of a physician, they are licensed to practice certain functions of medicine, such as prescribing medications and ordering tests. In many cases, a patient may only see a PA in the initial screening, or in the case of minor medical problems, such as the flu or a cold.

Medical assistants receive more direct supervision from doctors, nurses, and physician assistants. They are not licensed to practice medicine and cannot make independent assessments or diagnoses of patients. Nevertheless, their duties are wide ranging. They include both administrative and clinical tasks, from making appointments and organizing medical histories, to recording basic vital signs and performing basic laboratory tests.

Because of their versatility and enhanced training in recent years, medical assistants are becoming the allied health professionals of choice for a variety of healthcare settings. Medical assistants are members of a well-established profession and are in demand. An added benefit is that the typical training program requires only one- to two-years. There are also varied employment opportunities in addition to private practice, for example, in hospital departments, clinics, pharmacies, insurance companies, long-term care facilities, and other healthcare settings.

This report will help you learn more about the career, from specific job duties and educational requirements, to the observations of medical assistants currently on the job. If you are looking for an important, exciting healthcare career, and like working with a wide variety of people, certified medical assistant may be the right choice for you.

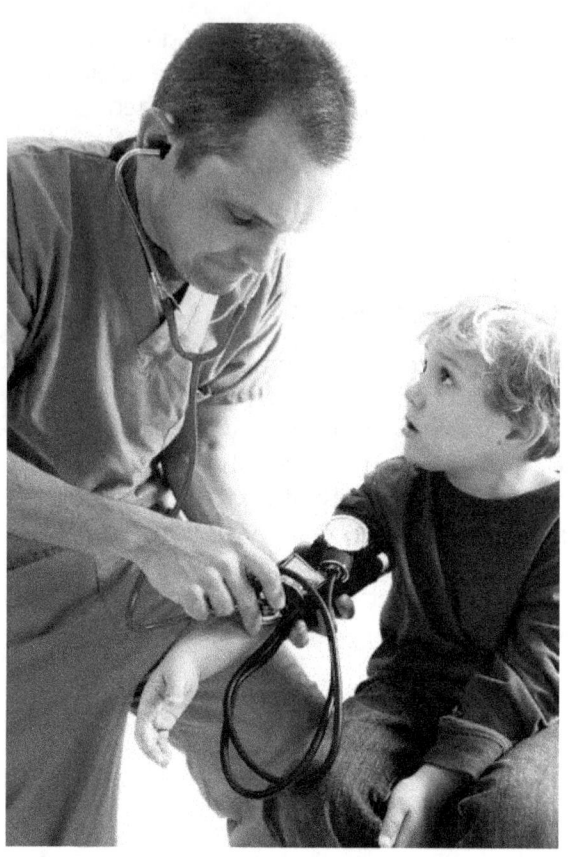

## WHAT YOU CAN DO NOW

THE FIRST STEP IN CHOOSING A CAREER is learning as much about that career as possible. This report is a good place to start since it provides a wide range of information including resources for more research you can do, including a list of medical assistant associations and websites. The American Association of Medical Assistants (AAMA), for example, includes on its website a list of local chapters of medical assistant societies, as well as state and local websites and social media pages, if available.

To help determine whether a healthcare career is right for you, volunteer in a medical setting, such as a hospital or clinic. The experience will give you a first-hand look at healthcare and what it is like to work with patients who are ill, disabled, and sometimes frightened. Volunteering also allows you to add this experience to your résumé and application for school or a training program. In addition to doctor's offices and clinics, there are volunteer opportunities in nursing homes, nurse associations, hospices, and hospitals. The American Red Cross also offers volunteer opportunities for students.

Ask yourself some important questions. Do you like working with people? Do you want to work in an office environment? Do you work well under supervision? Do you get along with a wide range of people, including patients from various socioeconomic and ethnic backgrounds, and fellow workers at different professional levels? Are you good at multitasking? Are you looking for variety in a career?

Because most physician offices or clinics now employ medical assistants, you can contact your doctor or a local clinic and see if it is possible to speak with a medical assistant first hand about the career. Ask them what the work is like, and find out what they like and dislike about their jobs.

If you are still in high school, talk with your guidance counselor about a career as a medical assistant. Investigate the potential training programs that are available in your area.

# HISTORY OF THE CAREER

THE DEVELOPMENT OF MEDICAL ASSISTANT as a profession is intertwined with the history of medical practice. For centuries, the physician was primarily a solitary practitioner who cared for patients on a one-on-one basis. These physicians did receive assistance, usually from members of the community, friends, and neighbors. Nevertheless, they practiced in simpler times with little medical technology, fewer therapeutic approaches to sickness and disease, and fewer rules and regulations providing oversight.

The beginnings of a more scientific and rigorous approach to medical care began in the 17th century, when physicians and scientists made important advances in understanding the biology of the human body. The following century saw a growing understanding of the reasons for many human diseases, such as the role bacteria play in causing diseases, from anthrax and cholera, to pneumonia and tetanus.

The 20th century was a time of phenomenal growth in the science of medicine, both in therapy and technology.

The economics of healthcare has also undergone dramatic changes. In the not too distant past, most patients simply paid on their own for any medical care they received, which was relatively inexpensive. Some doctors even bartered with their patients, accepting non-monetary payments for their services, such as food a farmer might grow, or some other items or services the patient might supply.

Today, with the rapidly rising cost of medical technology and procedures, and insurance coverage necessary to pay for expensive medical bills, new economics control how care is provided. As medical care became more complex, physicians found they could no longer practice in isolation. Insurance billing, government regulations, and the potential for lawsuits, required trained and dedicated support staff. This has become even truer today, where a rapidly aging baby-boom population that was born after World War II significantly impacts physician practices and healthcare economics.

The earliest use of the term "medical assistant" can be traced back to an 1883 court case when it was used to distinguish the duties of a doctor and of his helper involved in the case. By the 1950s, many physicians had "assistants." Although there was no required training for these aides, a New York City high school biology teacher named M. M. Mandl set up a school in 1924 to train students to work in physician offices. As an educator, Mandl realized that a strong educational program was needed to provide the intellectual training necessary for these assistants to function at a high level.

Mandl's school focused on training people in routine medical procedures, medical equipment operation, and office management. The goal was to enable graduates to help in medical, clinical and office environments, thus freeing physicians to devote more time to their patients.

By the 1950s, people working as assistants to doctors began to organize into professional groups. In 1955, a society of medical assistants in Kansas hosted 78 medical assistants from 15 other state societies to establish a national organization, which would be called the American Association of Medical Assistants (AAMA). Over the following two decades, the AAMA focused on establishing the medical assistant profession, through training and certification programs. By 1969, the AAMA had begun issuing accreditation for medical assistants, firmly establishing medical assistants as recognized professionals in the healthcare field. In 1974, the US Department of Education formally recognized a partnership between the American Medical Association's Council on Medical Education and the AAMA Program Approval Committee. This partnership formed an official accrediting agency for post-high school medical assisting programs. Medical assistants were formally recognized as allied health professionals.

Since that time, the medical assistant profession has burgeoned as doctor's offices and clinics are turning to this profession to run effective and efficient practices. The field's recognition among healthcare professionals and beyond has been so well established that in 2002 a certified medical assistant (CMA) pin traveled onboard the NASA Space Shuttle.

As the complexity of providing healthcare continues to increase, medical assistants will play an increasingly important role. New technologies, delivery systems, and approaches to facilitating cost-efficient and quality healthcare are all positive factors in the growing demand for medical assistants.

## WHERE YOU WILL WORK

MEDICAL ASSISTANTS WORK PRIMARILY in ambulatory patient settings, with about two thirds of all medical assistants employed in physician offices. The types of offices vary widely, from general practitioners to specialists in areas such as orthopedic surgery, otolaryngology, ophthalmology, and geriatric medicine. Medical assistants also work for podiatrists, chiropractors, and other healthcare providers.

Medical assistants may work in a group practice, and opportunities are available in clinics, health maintenance organizations (HMOs), occupational health centers, long-term care facilities, and hospitals. Other employers include medical supply businesses, home health agencies, and insurance companies.

About 15 percent of medical assistants work in public and private hospitals, including outpatient facilities, and another 10 percent work in offices of chiropractors, optometrists, podiatrists, and other healthcare practitioners.

It is important to remember that the work environment in a physician's office or clinic can vary, from tranquil to hectic, depending on factors such as the workload. The type of environment will largely depend on the staff that help make an office run smoothly. Overall, however, expect your working environment to be fast paced.

Medical assistants work in well lighted, clean, and comfortable general office environments and examination rooms. In some cases, they also work in laboratories.

Job opportunities for this field exist throughout the United States, from large metropolitan areas to rural areas and smaller towns. Although the availability of medical assistant jobs varies from city to city, the overall demand is strong throughout the United States. There are also opportunities overseas, working in physician offices, clinics, and hospitals. Volunteer work is available through organizations such as the Peace Corps and other medical aid organizations.

The US military employs medical assistants. They work in a military hospital or clinic in the United States or abroad, on land or aboard ships, as well as in mobile field hospitals near combat units. Some also work on cargo aircraft and are responsible for transporting wounded soldiers to a military hospital. The military offers a good training ground for a subsequent civilian career because military medical assistants typically have more responsibilities and independence than civilian counterparts, and therefore learn more on the job.

# DESCRIPTION OF WORK DUTIES

CERTIFIED MEDICAL ASSISTANTS ARE integral members of the healthcare team and have become critical front-line workers in the offices of physicians and clinics throughout the United States. Medical assistants are the closest match to registered nurses in abilities, as compared to other allied health occupations.

Qualified by education and experience, duties of CMAs are wide ranging and include administrative office, examination room, and laboratory work. As a liaison between the doctor and patient, the CMA is vitally important to a medical practice's success as doctors rely more and more on CMAs to gather information, consult with patients, and deal with a wide variety of office and medical issues.

A CMA's typical workday is varied and may include everything from making appointments over the telephone and greeting patients in the office, to taking patients' vital signs and doing lab procedures. Overall, duties vary depending on individual state laws and guidelines for CMAs, the size of the office, and specialization in a particular area, such as general medicine, ophthalmology, or podiatry. For example, in some states, CMAs can perform routine procedures such as urinalysis, blood pressure and weight checks, electrocardiograms, strep tests, and even venipuncture and injections.

In smaller offices, CMAs work as generalists who have office and clinical duties, as well as laboratory duties if the practice requires it. In most cases, the CMA reports directly to the physicians, nurses, other health practitioners, or office managers. In larger offices and practices, CMAs typically specialize in a particular area, administrative or clinical, for example.

In most cases, the physicians assess a CMA's skills and capabilities as they consider liability risk and quality control. Physicians provide direct supervision in most clinical cases.

Additional supervision is provided by nurse managers, to coordinate and maximize workflow.

Entry-level CMAs have a wide range of general duties that may include explaining treatment procedures to patients, and patient education. They typically help patients from diverse cultural backgrounds, acting as a patient advocate. They assist patients who may have physical or mental disabilities, or hearing or vision impairments. They also typically maintain medical records.

CMA duties can expand with experience and training. With experience, CMAs may be able to perform such advanced duties as office practice management, which may include strategic planning, as well as marketing and financial duties.

## Administrative Duties

On the administrative side, entry-level duties include greeting patients, handling correspondence, scheduling appointments, and answering the phones. Additional duties may include creating and maintaining medical records, performing medical transcription services, and arranging for hospital admissions. Medical assistants generally are also involved in billing procedures, bookkeeping, and insurance processing.

With experience comes advanced administrative duties, from developing and conducting public outreach programs to designing and maintaining fee schedules. Advanced CMAs may help negotiate equipment leasing and supply contracts, manage business and professional insurance, and work as a Health Information Portability and Accountability Act (HIPAA) compliance officer to ensure the protection of patients' personal health information. Negotiating non-risk and risk managed care contracts is another duty often given to advanced CMAs.

With even more experience comes the opportunity to

participate in practice analysis, which includes coordinating efforts to improve the overall practice, including expansion or consolidation issues. Duties may include personnel supervision – the hiring, training, and firing of employees; conducting performance reviews; maintaining personnel records; and acting as a leader and motivator of employees.

Information systems management duties may include managing spreadsheets and databases, as well as websites and email systems. CMAs may create computer presentations and graphics, and help prepare manuscripts and abstracts. Another duty is reviewing scientific and educational publications.

Advanced CMAs may perform various accounting duties, such as processing payroll and maintaining records. They may forecast and track capital expenditures and help with office budgets. They are often involved in preparing income projections and tax returns, and managing accounts payable and receivable.


## Clinical Duties

On the clinical side, entry-level CMAs may assist the physician during examinations and perform basic diagnostic tests, such as electrocardiograms and spirometry. Some states allow CMAs to give injections and perform phlebotomies, including venipuncture and capillary puncture. Other direct patient care duties include preparing patients for an examination and various tests, performing first aid and cardiopulmonary resuscitation, recording vital signs, taking medical histories, and removing sutures or changing dressing on wounds. They may also instruct patients about their medical care such as medication use and special diets, and teach patients about procedures prior to tests.

Entry-level CMAs are often responsible for infection control and asepsis, that is, ensuring the examination room and laboratory are free from disease causing contaminants such as bacteria, fungi, viruses, and parasites. They may also be responsible for disposing of contaminated supplies and sterilizing medical instruments. In addition, they usually call or email prescriptions in to pharmacies.

Advanced clinical duties may include initiating an intravenous (IV) therapy, including administering IV medications. These CMAs report diagnostic study results and help patients with establishing advanced directives and living wills concerning their medical care. With the proper training, they may also assist physicians in clinical trials.

CMAs are uniquely qualified to serve as a communication liaison between the busy physician and the patients. CMAs are patient advocates and health coaches. In this role they recognize and respect cultural diversity and communicate on a level patients can understand if they have questions about physician orders, a procedure, or medication. For example, if a doctor orders a patient to lose weight, the CMA works with the patient to draw up a dietary plan and helps teach the patient how to follow the plan. In all cases, CMAs use professional telephone and interpersonal techniques, and respond effectively to verbal, nonverbal, and written communications. This role also includes identifying the basics of office emergency preparedness.

## Laboratory Duties

The typical office or clinic laboratory is a facility that does laboratory testing on specimens from patients for information relevant to the diagnosis, prevention, and treatment of disease. In general, CMAs who have these duties may arrange laboratory services and collect, prepare, and transmit specimens. In addition, they typically instruct patients in how to collect specific specimens when required.

CMAs working in laboratories must oversee the general

performance in clinical laboratory tasks as regulated by law and the protocols within a particular medical practice. Laboratory CMAs are concerned with issues such as quality improvement, safety, procedural accuracy, and the regulatory practice standards that ensure a safe and effective laboratory operation. With appropriate training and certification, CMAs may also perform certain laboratory tests independently.

An important duty performed by some CMAs is ensuring adherence to the Clinical Laboratory Improvement Amendments (CLIA), a set of quality standards passed by the US Congress in 1988 for all laboratory testing, to ensure accuracy, reliability, and timeliness. For example, the CMA may be responsible for monitoring the temperature of specimens in storage to ensure their continued viability. CMAs also make certain that the laboratory is meeting the safety standards of laboratory work as outlined in the Occupational Safety and Health Administration (OSHA) guidelines. In some cases they serve as the OSHA compliance officer.

## Tools and Technology

CMAs also work with tools and technology associated with patient care. They prepare needles for injections, including intradermal needles, intramuscular needles, and subcutaneous hypodermic needles. They operate blood pressure units, as well as spirometers, which are apparatuses for measuring the volume of air inspired and expired by the lungs. Other technical equipment handled by CMAs include ophthalmoscopes (the familiar ophthalmologist's tool used to look inside a patient's eye), and otoscopes (a device used to look in patients' ears).

They are also trained to use the computer software relied on by every medical practice. For example, many physicians use electronic prescribing tools to send prescriptions to pharmacies. In many practices, medical records are accessible by patients online.

## Specialization

Some CMAs go on to specialize in a specific area of healthcare or administration. For example, they can train to work in orthopedics, optometry, podiatry, geriatrics, pediatrics, oncology, or numerous other medical specializations. They may also choose to focus on administration, including areas such as medical coding and billing.

For example, CMAs who specialize in optometry typically have fewer clinical duties than CMAs in other types of practices. Instead, they not only handle typical administrative duties but also perform basic eye exams and help prepare patients for surgical procedures. If they work in podiatry, they may help podiatrists make castings of feet, wash feet and cut toenails, apply dressings and bandages to feet, and develop and file x-rays. Medical coders, do not work directly with patients but instead abstract critical information from patients' records. They have expertise in reimbursement procedures and coding guidelines to maximize payments to the physician.

Much of the work is hands-on and no CMA has to worry about not having anything to do. The work duties are so varied that boring is rarely a word used to describe a medical assistant's day.

# CMAs TELL THEIR OWN STORIES

## I Am a Certified Medical Assistant

"I decided on a career as a medical assistant after I was laid off from my previous job. Initially, I was interested in a career as a medical transcriptionist but after going for an interview at the school, I was told that my background in the insurance business made me an ideal candidate to become a medical assistant. They also told me that graduates of the program were not having trouble finding jobs in my area. I did a little more research about the field on my own and decided that it was a good career choice for me. I like working with people and this seemed to offer a lot of variety in duties and responsibilities.

I was also pleased to find in my research that medical assistants are becoming more valued by physicians and nurses. I had heard that working with doctors can be demanding, and I had already been in jobs where my employer didn't seem to respect me. I happened to be acquainted with several doctors because of my work in the insurance industry. So, I called them to see what they thought of medical assistants. They told me that they couldn't imagine operating their practices without one, and that they were really important for helping with patient counseling, information gathering, and overall office work.

I now work for a medium size family practice clinic where my positive experience has lived up to everything I thought my career might entail. I schedule appointments, greet patients, take vital signs, give patients shots, order supplies and equipment, and also do some lab work. I am especially helpful in working with insurance carriers, since I know how they operate.

Most of all, I enjoy the relationships I have developed with our clinic's older patients. Sometimes they seem to be intimated by our doctors and are more willing to ask me questions. Most of our patients love me, which I attribute to the fact that I have more time than the doctors to sit and listen to them and thoroughly explain their test results and the doctor's orders.

On the other hand, my biggest headache is that sometimes I have to deal with difficult patients. It is my job to help calm them down and discuss issues that the doctors just don't have much time to deal with. For example, one elderly patient had a very negative view of the medical profession, and the patient kept questioning why the doctor ordered this test or prescribed a certain drug. I just stayed calm and took the time to explain the test results and why the patient definitely needed to follow the doctor's orders.

I think the fact that our patients see how well we all work together as a team in the clinic also bolsters my credibility with the patients. The physicians treat me with respect, and I think the patients pick up on that. Right now I'm thinking about going back to school to become a physician assistant, so I can do more on the clinical side of the practice. Because of my experience as a medical assistant, I think I'll have an advantage over people who are going into programs straight out of high school."

# I Am a Medical Assistant Student

"I'm a single mom who was looking for a secure and rewarding career that would allow me to work a normal nine-to-five job instead of my other two jobs working as a waitress and in a convenience store. I learned about medical assistants when one of my children had the flu and I took him to the doctor. I began talking with the person taking my son's blood pressure and asked how she liked being a nurse. She told me she wasn't a nurse but a medical assistant, and that she loved her job.

After asking her a few more questions, I was intrigued. I must admit that I was most attracted to the field when I learned that I could complete training in one to two years. I opted for the two-year associate degree program, and I am currently in the final stages of my training. I've finished courses in anatomy and physiology, clinical procedures, medical terminology, medical billing and coding, and law and ethics – which I found fascinating. Right now I'm doing my externship. Although I enjoyed learning about the human body and most of my classes overall, the externship is the best by far. The experience has been wonderful and has given me confidence that I can do this job.

The program at my technical college is really good. The teachers have been excellent and they seem to have numerous contacts with the community. One teacher has already recommended several places for me to apply for a job after I get my certification. The learning curve is intense but not overwhelming, especially if you are committed to the program.

I think it's important for potential students to know that my fellow students come from a wide variety of backgrounds. They vary in age from 18, right out of high school, to one man who is in his 50s and looking for a new career after losing his office job when the company closed. In fact, I was surprised to see that there were so many men in the program.

Although I had to take out loans to pay for my education, I am confident that it's all been worth it, you know, taking care of the kids, working a part-time job, studying late at night. I know the school is providing me with real skills to work in the real world.

Although studying to become a medical assistant is much easier than schooling to become a doctor or a nurse, you still need perseverance. Some of the courses were tougher than I thought they would be. The demands on my time going to class and doing homework until late at night, led me to consider dropping out at one point. I talked to one of my teachers about it, and she was very supportive and gave me some tips on how to better manage my time. She also gave me some studying tips as well.

Right now, I can't wait to graduate and get started. I'm already looking at places to apply, and my children promised to throw me a party at our local pizza place when I'm finished with school!"

## I Work for Chiropractors

"I chose to work in a chiropractic clinic because I suffered from back problems for many years and finally went to a chiropractor who told me my problems were muscular. Although he performed adjustments on me, he emphasized that I needed to do a series of stretching exercises more than anything else. After following my chiropractor's instructions, my back became less and less of a problem.

I also like the fact that chiropractors seem to take a more holistic approach than many medical doctors. They do not rely solely on medications to help their patients. Our chiropractors are well versed in the benefits of a wide range of therapies, such as nutrition and massage therapy. I also like that we focus on the prevention of problems as much as curing them.

I ended up getting hired by the clinic where I did my externship. I arrange patients' appointments and also handle insurance and patients' accounts. I really enjoy educating patients about chiropractic care and what to expect.

What I like best about my job, is that I have gained so much knowledge about getting and staying healthy. My job has definitely made me a healthier person and has dramatically changed my life. It's been very enjoyable working in the clinic and sharing knowledge about health and healing with our patients. I enjoy spreading the word about the benefits of chiropractic treatment to nonbelievers."

## I Work in a Hospital

"Although the majority of medical assistants work in private practices, I've always been interested in working for a hospital and jumped at the opportunity when it came up. I am not part of one department but rather work in various different departments depending on the hospital's needs at the time. Most of my duties involve hands-on care of patients, and each department has its own routines and needs. For example, the emergency department tends to be very hectic, while obstetrics seems, at least to me, to be a lot more laid back.

My typical day starts with a review of patients' charts, and then I take vitals on all the patients assigned to me. My duties include helping prepare patients for their meals, and I monitor everything the patients eat and drink. Once I compile this information, I forward it to the nurses on staff. Each department has its own specific duties. For example, in the obstetrics department I help feed the infants and transport them whenever needed. When I work in rehabilitation, I work alongside physical and occupational therapists, and help patients complete their rehabilitation exercises so they can ultimately return home.

Generally, however, my duties are very similar to someone working in a clinic. I help physicians and other clinical staff with general patient care, including preparing patients for examinations, taking vital signs, and posting surgical cases. I also help the medical office specialist with obtaining insurance authorization for surgery. I do not do filing, but I do answer the telephone sometimes and also schedule appointments under the direction of the business operations manager.

I should note that it is unusual for hospitals to hire medical assistants right out of school. Most prefer that their medical assistants have at least a few years of experience working in a clinic or some other private practice. The reason is that hospital patients tend to have more serious medical issues than those visiting their primary care physician. Certification is definitely a plus if you want to work in a hospital.

Although I worked for three years in a private practice, I think I landed my current position because I'm bilingual. We have a large Mexican population here and the fact that I'm fluent in Spanish was a real plus for me since I can communicate clearly with patients with little or no English skills. In addition, I am certified in CPR (cardiopulmonary resuscitation).

The one thing I can say for certain about working in a hospital is that you need to be able to work under pressure and adapt to a wide variety of medical situations. One advantage that medical assistants working in a private practice have is that they normally work Monday through Friday from 9 to 5. I have to work weekends and some holidays, as well as different shifts occasionally.

Still, I love my job. I like a challenge and constantly having new experiences. I also like working with many different kinds of people, both patients as well as doctors and nurses. Day in and day out, I am helping people. I honestly look forward to going to work."

## PERSONAL QUALIFICATIONS

MEDICAL ASSISTANTS MUST ENJOY working with all types of people. They are empathetic to the problems and concerns of others, especially patients who may be ill and frightened. They are active listeners who can give someone their full attention, and they have a certain instinct and perception that enables them to understand the reactions of patients and treat them with courtesy and tact.

Good communications skills are a standard requirement for all medical professionals. Medical assistants must be able to convey information effectively, both speaking and in written form. They have excellent reading comprehension. Because medical assistants work with people and are privy to sensitive information, they should have integrity and honesty, both to protect privacy and to ensure they provide the best service possible.

Critical thinking is important – using logic and reasoning to identify the best approaches and solutions to a problem. Other related skills are the ability to quickly evaluate a patient's circumstances and then begin taking the necessary action to help the patient. Critical thinking also comes into play when prioritizing work, especially important for medical assistants whose duties are often varied and fast moving. Critical thinking abilities can be improved over time as a medical assistant learns more on the job.

Paying attention to detail is essential. Whether administering drugs, completing patients' charts, or processing bills and insurance forms, the CMA must be totally accurate. For example, calling in a patient's prescription to the pharmacy, or administering a shot or other medication, must be done with upmost precision. Reliability is a hallmark of successful medical assistants. Physicians count on them for the unfailing provision of superior care.

Because the large majority of medical assistants have both administrative and clinical duties that are wide ranging, time management is an important skill. Good time management skills enable a CMA to function efficiently in a medical office, even when the pressure is great. It also helps reduce work stress.

CMA duties require flexibility because the medical assistant encounters a constant flow of new people and situations almost every day. A good positive attitude is also important, especially when dealing with patients. That means a positive, caring approach, taking direction from authority without questioning or complaint, and the ability to respond to criticism and see it as a learning experience.

A willingness to learn is essential in all healthcare. Just as physicians and nurses must continually study the latest advances in medical science and patient care, the CMA must keep up-to-date on technical and patient care issues, and be able to apply new knowledge to the job. For example, if you work with an oncologist, you might be asked to take a continuing education class on the latest advances in cancer care.

Certain physical requirements are integral to working as a medical assistant. There is some physical effort associated with the job so a CMA should be in relatively good health. Other traits such as manual dexterity, mobility, and good vision may also be required for performing tests and working in a technical environment.

## ATTRACTIVE FEATURES

WORKING AS A MEDICAL ASSISTANT IS A personally rewarding career. You get to meet and help people who really appreciate your efforts. You also work with professional healthcare providers who have the common goal of helping patients. In addition, CMAs are well respected by their employers, as well as within the general community.

A career in medical assisting offers versatility in daily work duties. In just one day, you may help prepare patients for examination, instruct them in how to follow doctor's orders, and prepare and administer medications under physician supervision. You may also answer phones, arrange appointments, record important patient and office data, and more.

Medical assisting is an expanding field that is becoming more and more essential to physicians. As a result, medical assistants enjoy stable job opportunities. On the other hand, becoming a medical assistant does not require the extensive education that many other healthcare professionals must pursue.

There are numerous career advancement opportunities gained through further studies, training, and experience. It is not uncommon for an experienced medical assistant to eventually consider furthering their education and expanding their career options, becoming a physician's assistant or a registered nurse, for example.

Most medical assistants have regular office or clinic hours and typically work 40 hours a week. They enjoy benefits such as paid vacations and holidays, as well as sick days and good insurance plans.

## UNATTRACTIVE FEATURES

WORKING AS A MEDICAL ASSISTANT can be very stressful for some people. They must attend to the needs of the physicians, the patients, and the office staff. Some may find such multiple tasks to be taxing and confusing.

Medical assistants are frequently exposed to communicable diseases from patients who, for example, may be suffering from a cold or the flu. Although this exposure typically comes via direct patient contact, it also may occur with exposure to specimens, body fluids, and wastes. Although the office and clinic environment is generally clean and safe, there are electrical and mechanical dangers. In addition, laboratory testing procedures may cause exposure to hazardous chemicals and specimens. Fortunately, protection and safety for the medical assistant comes in the form of personal protective equipment, such as gloves, face shields, and goggles.

The typical physician office or clinic is a hectic place, and being a medical assistant can be tiring. Not all patients are going to be understanding and considerate. Some will be in a bad mood (as may be expected when they are sick) – unreasonable and demanding.

Doctors and nurses can be set in their ways. Since they often directly supervise the medical assistant, this may cause problems. Veterans who have been doing things their own way for many years may not always welcome feedback from a CMA on how an office is functioning and how to improve it.

## EDUCATION AND TRAINING

TECHNICALLY, NO FORMAL TRAINING IS required to become a medical assistant other than a high school diploma. Realistically, the growing complexity of medical care, as well as the expanding practices of physicians and clinics, have resulted in physicians hiring better-trained candidates for their practice. In addition, more states are requiring medical assistants to take a test or attend a training program before they can perform certain job duties, especially those duties associated with clinical care.

As a result, formal training is highly desirable by employers who want their medical assistants to perform the entire scope of a medical assistant's possible duties. In addition, employers are increasingly requiring their medical assistants to pass a national certification examination demonstrating certain standards of competence.

A variety of medical assistant training programs are available throughout the United States. These programs provide training in clinical procedures, medical terminology, laboratory techniques, and record keeping. They also typically offer the opportunity for specialization in fields such as optometry and podiatry. Formal training provides graduates with a professional edge, increased job security, and higher prestige among colleagues.

Preference is usually given to graduates of an accredited medical assisting program offered by vocational schools, junior colleges, and colleges and universities. There are two accrediting agencies: the Commission on Accreditation of Allied Health Education Programs (CAAHEP) and the Accreditation Bureau of Health Education Schools (ABHES). Before choosing a program, it is important to determine that it is accredited. There are almost 600 medical assisting programs accredited by the CAAHEP and approximately 250 on the ABHES list.

Medical assistant training programs are one to two years in duration. They offer an associate degree, certificate, or diploma. The only prerequisite for entering a program is a high school diploma or equivalent, such as passing the General Educational Development (GED) test. Generally, degree and certificate programs focus on specialized knowledge directly related to the work, while diploma programs provide a more comprehensive education that may include courses in English, speech, math, and communications.

Although the curriculum may vary, most training programs include classes in anatomy and physiology, psychology, medical terminology, administrative procedures, accounting practices, clinical and diagnostic procedures, laboratory techniques, pharmacology, first aid, insurance procedures, and patient relations. Training programs also include instruction in performing EKGs, urinalysis, phlebotomy, injections, assisting with minor surgery, wound care, eye and ear irrigation, casting, urinary catheterization, and other hands-on clinical training. Training programs typically require students to complete an externship that provides practical experience in physicians' offices, hospitals, or other care facilities.

## Certification

The American Association of Medical Assistants awards the Certified Medical Assistant (CMA) credential, which is the best recognized in the field.

There are several other possibilities. The American Medical Technologists organization confers the Registered Medical Assistant (RMA) credential. The National Certified Medical Assistant (NCMA) is offered by the National Center for Competency Testing, and the Certified Clinical Medical Assistant (CCMA) is available from the National Health Career Association.

In areas of specialization, other associations also offer certification, such as the American Society of Podiatric Medical Assistants and the Joint Commission on Allied Health in Ophthalmology.

Although some high schools provide the courses necessary to begin a career as a medical assistant, certification without formal training is not possible until a medical assistant has five years of experience. Certification requires an exam. Once certified, a medical assistant must be recertified every five years. This is attained either by taking continuing education credits or a new certification test.

Professionals with formal education have the best job prospects. In addition, certified medical assistants have more opportunities for advancement in their careers. Certification shows that the medical assistant is knowledgeable in the field, and it looks good on the résumé.

## Paying for Training

The costs of attending a medical assistant program vary, but typically range from about $2,000 to $4,000 at vocational training schools offering one-year programs. However, that can increase with degree programs, which can sometimes cost $10,000 or more.

Financial aid is available for most programs but not all, so this is something a prospective student should investigate before applying. Typical aid programs include Federal Pell Grants (which do not have to be repaid), Federal Supplemental Educational Opportunity Grants, Federal Direct Subsidized Stafford Loans, Federal Direct PLUS Loans (made to the parents), Federal Perkins Loans, and scholarships such as the medical assistant scholarship offered by the American Medical Technologists (AMT) organization.

Before seeking financial assistance from the federal government, it is a good idea to fill out the Free Application for Federal Student Aid (FAFSA) for students seeking to attend college or a career school. To find out if you qualify for federal financial aid, visit the FAFSA website at http://www.fafsa.ed.gov. You will find information on filing options and deadlines.

## EARNINGS

THERE ARE SEVERAL VARIABLES THAT affect how much a medical assistant earns. Experience and skill level are important factors, as is educational background. Overall, CMAs make more annually than non-certified medical assistants, with CMAs earning an average of more than $3,000 above those with no certification. Salaries increase with experience. With less than two years' experience, earnings average about $25,000 annually. Those with 10 years of experience can expect $30,000, and those with 15 years or more of experience reach $35,000.

Where the medical assistant works also affects earnings. Those working in a physician office earn somewhat more than those in other types of medical practices. Hospitals pay even more. CMAs working in higher education report that they earn at least $50,000 annually.

Scientific research and development services pay certified medical assistants an annual salary of $40,000, but there are not many employed in that specialty.

Another factor to consider is geographic location. For example, medical assistants working in Alaska earn about $40,000. Other states with generally higher salaries include Massachusetts, Hawaii, and Washington, as well as the District of Columbia. On the other end of the spectrum, medical assistants working in Alabama may earn only about $25,000 a year, while those working in West Virginia may earn as little as $24,000 a year.

Yet another factor in earnings is whether a medical assistant works in a large metropolitan area. Medical assistants are likely to make more working in a large city such as Fairbanks, Alaska ($45,000) or San Francisco, California ($42,000).

Remember that the cost of living in some states and metropolitan areas is a major factor in pay. For example, the cost of living in Alaska or Hawaii is much higher than in West Virginia or Alabama. This means that food, housing, gas, and many other items typically cost more.

## Benefits

Medical assistants typically have good benefits that help supplement their earnings. In addition to paid vacations and sick leave, medical assistants typically have access to good health and vision insurance plans that are paid in part by their employers. Dental and vision insurance is also common, especially for medical assistants who work in these specialties. Another insurance benefit may include a long--term-disability and accident plan.

Many employers also offer pension and retirement plans. Especially when the employers are larger clinics or institutions, retirement matching plans are available, in which employers match the contributions their employees make. Working in a hospital or a clinic may include discounts when the medical assistant uses their medical services. In some cases, this discount may also apply to family members. Most employers also pay for all or some of continuing education classes to ensure that their medical assistants stay up-to-date in their field.

## OPPORTUNITIES

OPPORTUNITIES FOR MEDICAL ASSISTANTS are excellent, and the field is one of the fastest growing allied health careers. A number of factors are contributing to this growth, including an emphasis on cost-effective healthcare while ensuring quality patient care. Another factor is the rapidly growing elderly population in the United States, which means more and more people needing medical care. With expanded health insurance, Medicare, and Medicaid, these patients have better access to medical care.

Outpatient clinics and health maintenance organizations (HMOs) are on the rise as both the elderly and the overall population in the United States increases. In addition, the number of physicians joining large group practices is also increasing, meaning even more medical assistants and other support staff are needed. Certification programs for medical assistants have made these employees more valuable.

There were about 400,000 medical assistant jobs in the United States in 2006. By 2010, the number of positions increased to over 525,000 jobs. Experts predict that there will be a 30 percent growth rate over the next decade. Within that period, there will be as many as 200,000 new medical assistant jobs.

Medical assistants also have many opportunities for advancement. They can become office managers, clinical supervisors, or work in a variety of administrative positions. Many use their medical assistant training and experience as a stepping stone to other careers in healthcare. For example, they may obtain a bachelor's degree in an area such as human services or health services management. Some go on to receive further training to become a physician assistant, a medical technologist, or a nurse.

## GETTING STARTED

YOU CAN GET STARTED RIGHT NOW working toward your goal. For high school students, the most important thing is to focus on your classes. Because training programs to become a certified medical assistant include biology, chemistry, anatomy, and physiology courses, it is important to take full advantage of related courses in high school, as well as math. Since communications is a key aspect of the medical assistant's job, students should work hard in English and speech classes. CMAs also typically have administrative duties, so typing and other office management courses, including computers, should be included. It is also a good idea to talk to your school guidance counselor about the field and discuss possible training programs.

Medical assistants work in a variety of professional environments so you might want to begin considering where you would like to work. For example, you could work for a general practitioner, an optometrist, a chiropractor, or a podiatrist. You can work in a private practice, a clinic, or a hospital. Visiting these different settings and talking to professionals who work there can help you determine which environment suits you best.

Start looking for a school or training program to attend. Create a list of schools you are interested in attending and research them on the Internet. Contact the school and ask about the courses offered. Remember that not all programs are created equal. Look for programs that are well rounded and that offer a variety of clinical and administrative courses. They should also offer an externship that provides hands-on experience.

Determine whether the school is accredited. This is especially important for online programs. Remember, the demand is increasing at a much higher rate for those who are certified. If you do not have on-the-job experience, you can only become certified if you have graduated from an accredited program.

## ASSOCIATIONS

■ **American Association of Medical Assistants (AAMA)**
**http://www.aama-ntl.org**

■ **American Dental Assistant Association**
**http://www.dentalassistant.org**

■ **American Medical Technologists**
**http://www.americanmedtech**
**.org/default.aspx**

■ **American Society of Podiatric Medical Assistants**
**http://www.aspma.org**

■ **Commission on Accreditation of Allied Health Education Programs**
**http://www.caahep.org**

■ **Joint Commission on Allied Health Personal in Ophthalmology**
**http://www.jcahpo.org**

■ **American Society of Podiatric Medical Assistants**
**http://www.aspma.org**

# PUBLICATIONS

■ **Medical Assistant (Careers Without College Series)**

■ **CMA Today**
http://www.aama-ntl.org/CMAToday/about.aspx

# WEBSITES

■ **ABHES Online Directory**
https://ams.abhes.org/ams
/onlineDirectory/pages/directory.aspx
Search for programs accredited by the Accrediting Bureau of Health Education Schools

■ **Accredited Program Search – CAAHEP**
http://www.caahep.org/Find-An
-Accredited-Program

■ **Certified Medical Assistant.net**
www.CertifiedMedicalAssistant.net
News and articles about the profession, a job search page, and a listing of industry-related magazines

■ **Medical Assistant Net**
http://www.medicalassistant.net
Information on training programs, externships, certification, and job opportunities, as well as a medical assistant forum

www.ingramcontent.com/pod-product-compliance
Lightning Source LLC
Chambersburg PA
CBHW070747180526
45168CB00004B/1560